# the H(U)B

## BOOK

## FITNESS CENTERED AROUND [U]

# Luke Owens

### With foreword by Clay Clark

## Copyright Info

# Special Foreword by Clay Clark

### (Host of the iTunes chart-topping Thrive-TimeShow Podcast)

I grow businesses for a living and Luke Owens helps most people to shrink (to lose weight) for a living. Throughout these past years we have become friends, as a result of working together to grow The Hub Gym. As I have worked with Luke over the past three years to show him the practical steps needed to grow his business I have been shocked by how sincerely motivated he is to help YOU to get in the best shape of YOUR life. Almost to a fault, Luke's ENTIRE REASON for starting The Hub Gym was to help people like YOU regardless of whether his gym was profitable or not. Luke certainly did not start The Hub Gym for the love of money.

> "A friendship founded on business is better than a business founded on friendship."
> - John D. Rockefeller
> (The world's wealthiest man during his lifetime)

Despite having struggled for years without the knowledge of the proper marketing systems and processes, Luke never lost his passion for why he actually started The Hub Gym, his passion to help YOU. As the host of The Thrivetime Show Podcast, I've had the opportunity to personally interview America's business leaders, countless millionaires and billionaires who all achieved tremendous success in part because, much like Luke, they chose to NEVER lose their passion for their PURPOSE. As far as I'm concerned, Luke is at the top 1% of entrepreneurs when it comes to his passion for helping his customers and that's saying alot considering that I've been blessed with the opportunity to interview:

**Michael Levine** - The public relations consultant of choice for Nike, Prince, Michael Jackson, President Clinton and Charlton Heston

**Wolfgang Puck** - The man whose name has become synonymous with fine dining, Horst Schultz, the co-founder of Ritz-Carlton

**David Robinson** - The NBA Hall of Fame basketball player, turned successful investor and entrepreneur

**Scott Belsky** - The founder of Behance and the Chief Product Officer and Executive Vice President of Adobe

**John Maxwell** - The 8x New York Times best-selling author and leadership expert

**Guy Kawasaki** - The legendary former key Apple employee

turned venture capitalist and best selling author

**Sharon Lechter** - The New York Times best-selling co-author of *Rich Dad Poor Dad*

**Pastor Craig Groeschel** - The Senior pastor of the largest church in America with over 100,000 weekly attendees (Lifechurch.tv)

**David Bach** - One of America's most trusted financial experts and has written nine consecutive New York Times best-sellers with 7 million+ books in print

**Zack O'Malley Greenburg** - The senior editor for *Forbes* and 3x best-selling author

**John Lee Dumas** - The most downloaded business podcaster of all-time (EOFire.com)

**Seth Godin** - New York Times best-selling author of *Purple Cow*, and former Yahoo! vice president of marketing

**Dan Heath** - New York Times best-selling author of *Made to Stick* and Duke University Professor

**Lee Cockerell** - The former executive vice president of Walt Disney World who once managed 40,000 employees

**Ben Shapiro** - Conservative talk pundit, frequent Fox News contributor, political commentator and best-selling author

See additional guests at ThrivetimeShow.com

As you read this book know that Luke Owens is a **MANIACALLY OBSESSIVE** advocate for your personal health and overall wellness and that he is only writing this book to help provide you with both the practical steps and the inspiration needed to achieve your fitness goals. This is YOUR year to get in the best shape of your life and I believe that Luke and his team are the people you need in your life to help you to achieve your goals.

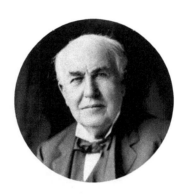

"Vision without execution is
hallucination."
- Thomas Edison
(The man who is credited with inventing the first
modern practical lightbulb, recorded sound and
recorded video, and the founder of General Electric)

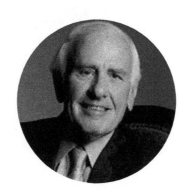

"You're the average of the five people
you spend the most time with."
- Jim Rohn
(Best-selling author and renowned speaker)

# Chapter 1
# CHALLENGE YOURSELF

"It does not matter how slowly you go as long as you do not stop."
- Confucius
(The Chinese teacher, politician, and philosopher. The philosophy of Confucius, also known a Confucianism which emphasizes personal morality, justice and sincerity.)

Hi, my name is Luke Owens and I'm the founder of The Hub Gym. I started this gym for YOU because I believe in your personal power and ability to change your habits, your lifestyle, and your waistline in as little as 30 days. If you simply follow the game plan in this book for the next 30 days you will lose weight, you will begin to gain personal momentum in your life and you will both feel and look better. However, if you simply read these words you will not get in better shape and I will have failed to achieve my goal, which is to help you to achieve your fitness goals.

Once You Commit to the Process You Will See Real Results

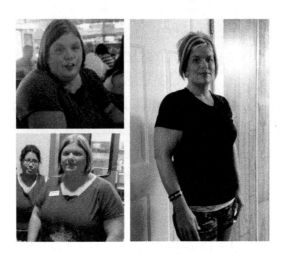

Tina W. - Transformation

"Change might not be fast and it isn't
always easy. But with time and effort,
almost any habit can be reshaped."
- Charles Duhigg
(The best selling author of *The Power of Habit: Why
We Do
What We Do in Life & Business*)

In our microwave society of instant gratification it's very
common for most people to jump from fitness fad to fitness
fad and from new diet to new diet in hopes of receiving
instant game-changing results. But in order to achieve success
in the world of fitness we have to change our habits, and it's
going to take you about 30 days to create a fat-burning habit.
Having worked with thousands of clients just like you, I also
know that changing a habit can be daunting which is why at

The Hub we do something different from most gyms you've ever been to. We call this the 30 Day Hub Habit-Changing Challenge, this challenge is designed to help every new member, and that includes you. Here's how it works.

YOU CAN EARN YOUR MONEY BACK!

If you will simply follow our game plan for the next 30 days you will not only lose the weight, but you will actually earn one month's membership fees 100% for free. In order to make sure that our challenge is super easy for everybody to implement, we have made our challenge simple and results focused. For the next 30 days you need to commit to only eating organic meat, vegetables, drinking water and to working out for 30 minutes per day three days per week. There are many scientific reasons behind why you want to do this, but at the end of the day if you will only eat organic meat, organic vegetables and drink water during the next 30 days your body is going to become a fat-burning machine, because it is sugar that causes us to get fat and not fat that causes your body to gain fat. Removing sugar from your diet will allow your body to address the inflammation which causes chronic pain and other health issues. Once you reduce the pain and inflammation you've been dealing with on a daily basis you will be able to move more freely and start your journey to health and fitness.

"The simple answer as to why we get fat is that carbohydrates make us so; protein and fat do not."
- Gary Taubes
(Best Selling Author of *Why We Get Fat*)

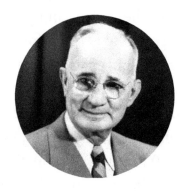

"The time will never be just right. You must act now."
- Napoleon Hill
(Best-selling author of *Think and Grow Rich*)

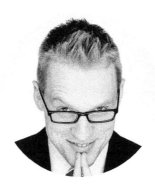

"When you implement proven systems,
processes and strategies you cannot lose."
- Clay Clark
(Host of the ThriveTimeShow.com podcast and
Oklahoma's former U.S. Small Business Administration
Entrepreneur of the Year)

# Chapter 2
## The Meal Plan

"If it didn't come from the ground or the ocean or have a mother—don't eat it. Think about it. Twinkies and Cheetos—what the hell are these? There's no Twinkie tree, and I'm pretty positive that nothing ever gave birth to a Cheeto."
- Jillian Michaels

(American personal trainer, businesswoman, author and television personality best known for being a trainer on the show *The Biggest Loser*.)

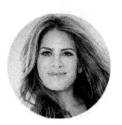

For the next 30 days, you must only consume organic meat, organic vegetables, and water. Don't make this weird or overly complicated, only eat organic meat, organic vegetables and drink water.

- What can you drink? Water.
- What can you eat? Organic meat and vegetables.

**Why?** Because the sugar, wheat, sweets and the sugary beverages that they serve at Starbucks are making you

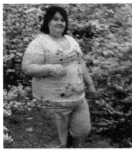
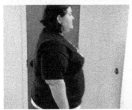
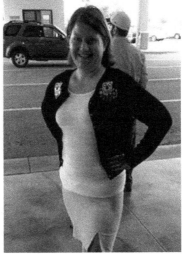

fat. You simply cannot out train a bad diet.

**Why? It's called insulin levels.**
So let's review. During the next 30 days in order to

*Krystal S. - Transformation*

achieve your fitness goals you can only consume organic meat, organic vegetables and drink water. Which means during the next 30 days you cannot eat wheat, sugar, drink alcohol, or drink pre-workout drinks, or anything that is not water or black coffee

What can I drink during the next 30 days?
Water or black coffee (no sugar or cream).

**What can I eat during the next 30 days?**
Organic meat and organic vegetables.

**What kind of meat can I eat?**
You can eat any kind of meat you want; you just need to ensure it is organic meat.

**What kind of vegetables can I eat?**
You can eat any kind of organic vegetables, and you can eat as much as you want.

**Day 1:**

Did you eat anything other than organic meat, vegetables and drink water? (Yes or No)

Did you work out? (Yes or No)

**Day 2:**

Did you eat anything other than organic meat, vegetables and drink water? (Yes or No)

Did you work out? (Yes or No)

**Day 3:**

Did you eat anything other than organic meat, vegetables and drink water? (Yes or No)

Did you work out? (Yes or No)

Once you've completed the 30 Day Hub Habit-Changing Challenge, simply turn your daily log into the front desk and we will credit your account with one free month; and as a byproduct you will also have developed the healthy-eating habits needed to get, and stay in, the best shape of your life.

# Day 1: Only eat organic meat, vegetables, and drink water

Meal 1

_____

_____

_____

_____

Meal 2

_____

_____

_____

_____

Meal 3

_____

_____

_____

_____

Meal 1

_____

_____

_____

_____

_____

_____

_____

_____

_____

_____

_____

_____

_____

_____

_____

_____

_____

| EXERCISE | SET #1 | SET #2 | SET #3 | SET #4 | SET #5 |
|---|---|---|---|---|---|
| Pulldowns - Wide Grip & Narrow Grip | x20 | x20 | x20 | x20 | |
| Seated Row | x15 | x15 | x15 | x15 | |
| Bent "Dumbbell" Row | x20 | x20 | x20 | x20 | |
| Machine Bicep Curl | x15 | x15 | x15 | | |
| Standing Barbell Curl | x10 | x10 | x10 | x10 | |
| Seated Alternating Dumbbell Curl | x20 | x20 | x20 | x20 | |

**30**DAY Challenge HUB Habit-Changing

Today's Date: _____ / _____ / _____

Meal 1

_____
_____
_____
_____

Meal 2

_____
_____
_____
_____

Meal 3

_____
_____
_____
_____

Meal 1

_____
_____
_____
_____
_____
_____
_____
_____
_____
_____
_____
_____
_____
_____
_____
_____
_____
_____
_____

# CARDIO FOR 45 MINUTES

**30**DAY HUB Habit-Changing Challenge

Today's Date: _____ / _____ / _____

**Day 3:** Only eat organic meat, vegetables, and drink water

Meal 1

_____
_____
_____
_____

Meal 2

_____
_____
_____
_____

Meal 3

_____
_____
_____
_____

Meal 1

_____
_____
_____
_____
_____
_____
_____
_____
_____
_____
_____
_____
_____
_____
_____
_____
_____
_____

| EXERCISE | SET #1 | SET #2 | SET #3 | SET #4 | SET #5 |
|---|---|---|---|---|---|
| Leg Extensions | | | | | |
| Squat | | | | | |
| Leg Press | | | | | |
| Leg Curl | | | | | |
| Lunge - Barbell/DB/Static/Step Up | | | | | |
| Leg Extensions | | | | | |

**30**DAY HUB Habit-Changing Challenge

Today's Date: _____ / _____ / _____

**Day 4:** Only eat organic meat, vegetables, and drink water

Meal 1

_____
_____
_____
_____

Meal 2

_____
_____
_____
_____

Meal 3

_____
_____
_____
_____

Meal 1

_____
_____
_____
_____
_____
_____
_____
_____
_____
_____
_____
_____
_____
_____
_____
_____
_____
_____
_____
_____
_____

# CARDIO FOR 45 MINUTES

**30**DAY HUB Habit-Changing Challenge

Today's Date: _____ / _____ / _____

**Day 5:** Only eat organic meat, vegetables, and drink water

Meal 1

_____
_____
_____
_____

Meal 2

_____
_____
_____
_____

Meal 3

_____
_____
_____
_____

Meal 1

_____
_____
_____
_____
_____
_____
_____
_____
_____
_____
_____
_____
_____
_____
_____
_____
_____

| EXERCISE | SET #1 | SET #2 | SET #3 | SET #4 |
|---|---|---|---|---|
| Incl. Flyes - Dumbbell | x10 | x10 | x10 | x10 |
| DB incline Bench Press | x10 | x10 | x10 | x10 |
| Machine Bench Press | x15 | x15 | x15 | x15 |
| Tricep "ARM" Extension | x15 | x15 | x15 | |
| Tricep Dumbbell Kickback | x20 | x20 | x20 | x20 |
| Overhead Press | x20 | x20 | x20 | x20 |
| Dumbbell Lateral Raises | x10 | x10 | x10 | x10 |
| Dumbbell Front Raise | x10 | x10 | x10 | x10 |
| High Pull | x10 | x10 | x10 | x10 |

**30**DAY HUB Habit-Changing Challenge

Today's Date: _____ / _____ / _____

**Day 6:** Only eat organic meat, vegetables, and drink water

Meal 1
_____
_____
_____
_____

Meal 2
_____
_____
_____
_____

Meal 3
_____
_____
_____
_____

Meal 1
_____
_____
_____
_____
_____
_____
_____
_____
_____
_____
_____
_____
_____
_____
_____
_____
_____
_____

# CARDIO FOR 45 MINUTES

**30**DAY HUB Habit-Changing Challenge

Today's Date: _____ / _____ / _____

# Day 7: Only eat organic meat, vegetables, and drink water

Meal 1

_____
_____
_____
_____

Meal 2

_____
_____
_____
_____

Meal 3

_____
_____
_____
_____

Meal 1

_____
_____
_____
_____
_____
_____
_____
_____
_____
_____
_____
_____
_____
_____
_____
_____
_____
_____
_____

| EXERCISE | SET #1 | SET #2 | SET #3 | SET #4 | SET #5 |
|---|---|---|---|---|---|
| Pulldowns - Wide Grip & Narrow Grip | x20 | x20 | x20 | x20 | |
| Seated Row | x15 | x15 | x15 | x15 | |
| Bent "Dumbbell" Row | x20 | x20 | x20 | x20 | |
| Machine Bicep Curl | x15 | x15 | x15 | | |
| Standing Barbell Curl | x10 | x10 | x10 | x10 | |
| Seated Alternating Dumbbell Curl | x20 | x20 | x20 | x20 | |

**30**DAY HUB Habit-Changing Challenge

Today's Date: _____ / _____ / _____

**Day 8:** Only eat organic meat, vegetables, and drink water

Meal 1

_____
_____
_____
_____

Meal 2

_____
_____
_____
_____

Meal 3

_____
_____
_____
_____

Meal 1

_____
_____
_____
_____
_____
_____
_____
_____
_____
_____
_____
_____
_____
_____
_____
_____
_____
_____
_____

# CARDIO FOR 45 MINUTES

**30**DAY HUB Habit-Changing Challenge

Today's Date: _____ / _____ / _____

# Day 9: Only eat organic meat, vegetables, and drink water

Meal 1

_____
_____
_____
_____

Meal 2

_____
_____
_____
_____

Meal 3

_____
_____
_____
_____

Meal 1

_____
_____
_____
_____
_____
_____
_____
_____
_____
_____
_____
_____
_____
_____
_____
_____
_____
_____

| EXERCISE | SET #1 | SET #2 | SET #3 | SET #4 | SET #5 |
|---|---|---|---|---|---|
| Leg Extensions | | | | | |
| Squat | | | | | |
| Leg Press | | | | | |
| Leg Curl | | | | | |
| Lunge - Barbell/DB/Static/Step Up | | | | | |
| Leg Extensions | | | | | |

**30**DAY HUB Habit-Changing Challenge

Today's Date: _____ / _____ / _____

**Day 9:** Only eat organic meat, vegetables, and drink water

Meal 1
_____
_____
_____
_____

Meal 2
_____
_____
_____
_____

Meal 3
_____
_____
_____
_____

Meal 1
_____
_____
_____
_____
_____
_____
_____
_____
_____
_____
_____
_____
_____
_____
_____
_____
_____

# CARDIO FOR 45 MINUTES

**30**DAY HUB Habit-Changing Challenge

Today's Date: _____ / _____ / _____

# Day 10: Only eat organic meat, vegetables, and drink water

Meal 1

_____
_____
_____
_____

Meal 2

_____
_____
_____
_____

Meal 3

_____
_____
_____
_____

Meal 1

_____
_____
_____
_____
_____
_____
_____
_____
_____
_____
_____
_____
_____
_____
_____
_____
_____
_____

| EXERCISE | SET #1 | SET #2 | SET #3 | SET #4 |
|---|---|---|---|---|
| Incl. Flyes - Dumbbell | x10 | x10 | x10 | x10 |
| DB incline Bench Press | x10 | x10 | x10 | x10 |
| Machine Bench Press | x15 | x15 | x15 | x15 |
| Tricep "ARM" Extension | x15 | x15 | x15 |  |
| Tricep Dumbbell Kickback | x20 | x20 | x20 | x20 |
| Overhead Press | x20 | x20 | x20 | x20 |
| Dumbbell Lateral Raises | x10 | x10 | x10 | x10 |
| Dumbbell Front Raise | x10 | x10 | x10 | x10 |
| High Pull | x10 | x10 | x10 | x10 |

**30**DAY HUB Habit-Changing Challenge

Today's Date: _____ / _____ / _____

# Day 11: Only eat organic meat, vegetables, and drink water

Meal 1

_____
_____
_____
_____

Meal 1

_____
_____
_____
_____
_____
_____
_____
_____

Meal 2

_____
_____
_____
_____

Meal 3

_____
_____
_____
_____

_____
_____
_____
_____
_____
_____
_____
_____
_____
_____
_____

# CARDIO FOR 45 MINUTES

**30**DAY HUB Habit-Changing Challenge

Today's Date: _____ / _____ / _____

# Day 12: Only eat organic meat, vegetables, and drink water

Meal 1

_____
_____
_____
_____

Meal 2

_____
_____
_____

Meal 3

_____
_____
_____
_____

Meal 1

_____
_____
_____
_____
_____
_____
_____
_____
_____
_____
_____
_____
_____
_____
_____
_____
_____
_____
_____

| EXERCISE | SET #1 | SET #2 | SET #3 | SET #4 | SET #5 |
|---|---|---|---|---|---|
| Pulldowns - Wide Grip & Narrow Grip | x20 | x20 | x20 | x20 | |
| Seated Row | x15 | x15 | x15 | x15 | |
| Bent "Dumbbell" Row | x20 | x20 | x20 | x20 | |
| Machine Bicep Curl | x15 | x15 | x15 | | |
| Standing Barbell Curl | x10 | x10 | x10 | x10 | |
| Seated Alternating Dumbbell Curl | x20 | x20 | x20 | x20 | |

**30**DAY HUB Habit-Changing Challenge

Today's Date: _____ / _____ / _____

Meal 1

_____
_____
_____
_____

Meal 2

_____
_____
_____
_____

Meal 3

_____
_____
_____
_____

Meal 1

_____
_____
_____
_____
_____
_____
_____
_____
_____
_____
_____
_____
_____
_____
_____
_____
_____
_____

# CARDIO FOR 45 MINUTES

**30**DAY HUB Habit-Changing Challenge

Today's Date: _____ / _____ / _____

# Day 14: Only eat organic meat, vegetables, and drink water

Meal 1

_____

_____

_____

_____

Meal 2

_____

_____

_____

_____

Meal 3

_____

_____

_____

_____

Meal 1

_____

_____

_____

_____

_____

_____

_____

_____

_____

_____

_____

_____

_____

_____

_____

_____

_____

_____

| EXERCISE | SET #1 | SET #2 | SET #3 | SET #4 | SET #5 |
|---|---|---|---|---|---|
| Leg Extensions | | | | | |
| Squat | | | | | |
| Leg Press | | | | | |
| Leg Curl | | | | | |
| Lunge - Barbell/DB/Static/Step Up | | | | | |
| Leg Extensions | | | | | |

**30**DAY HUB Habit-Changing Challenge

Today's Date: _____ / _____ / _____

**Day 15:** Only eat organic meat, vegetables, and drink water

Meal 1
_____
_____
_____
_____

Meal 2
_____
_____
_____
_____

Meal 3
_____
_____
_____
_____

Meal 1
_____
_____
_____
_____
_____
_____
_____
_____
_____
_____
_____
_____
_____
_____
_____
_____
_____
_____
_____
_____
_____
_____
_____

# CARDIO FOR 45 MINUTES

**30**DAY HUB Habit-Changing Challenge

Today's Date: _____ / _____ / _____

**Day 16:** Only eat organic meat, vegetables, and drink water

Meal 1

_____
_____
_____
_____

Meal 2

_____
_____
_____
_____

Meal 3

_____
_____
_____
_____

Meal 1

_____
_____
_____
_____
_____
_____
_____
_____
_____
_____
_____
_____
_____
_____
_____
_____
_____
_____
_____

| EXERCISE | SET #1 | SET #2 | SET #3 | SET #4 |
|---|---|---|---|---|
| Incl. Flyes - Dumbbell | x10 | x10 | x10 | x10 |
| DB incline Bench Press | x10 | x10 | x10 | x10 |
| Machine Bench Press | x15 | x15 | x15 | x15 |
| Tricep "ARM" Extension | x15 | x15 | x15 | |
| Tricep Dumbbell Kickback | x20 | x20 | x20 | x20 |
| Overhead Press | x20 | x20 | x20 | x20 |
| Dumbbell Lateral Raises | x10 | x10 | x10 | x10 |
| Dumbbell Front Raise | x10 | x10 | x10 | x10 |
| High Pull | x10 | x10 | x10 | x10 |

**30**DAY HUB Habit-Changing Challenge

Today's Date: _____ / _____ / _____

Meal 1
_____
_____
_____
_____

Meal 1
_____
_____
_____
_____
_____
_____
_____

Meal 2
_____
_____
_____
_____

_____
_____
_____
_____
_____
_____

Meal 3
_____
_____
_____
_____

_____
_____
_____
_____

# CARDIO FOR 45 MINUTES

**30**DAY HUB Habit-Changing Challenge

Today's Date: _____ / _____ / _____

# Day 18: Only eat organic meat, vegetables, and drink water

Meal 1
_____
_____
_____
_____

Meal 2
_____
_____
_____
_____

Meal 3
_____
_____
_____
_____

Meal 1
_____
_____
_____
_____
_____
_____
_____
_____
_____
_____
_____
_____
_____
_____
_____
_____
_____
_____

| EXERCISE | SET #1 | SET #2 | SET #3 | SET #4 | SET #5 |
|---|---|---|---|---|---|
| Pulldowns - Wide Grip & Narrow Grip | x20 | x20 | x20 | x20 | |
| Seated Row | x15 | x15 | x15 | x15 | |
| Bent "Dumbbell" Row | x20 | x20 | x20 | x20 | |
| Machine Bicep Curl | x15 | x15 | x15 | | |
| Standing Barbell Curl | x10 | x10 | x10 | x10 | |
| Seated Alternating Dumbbell Curl | x20 | x20 | x20 | x20 | |

**30**DAY HUB Habit-Changing Challenge

Today's Date: _____ / _____ / _____

**Day 19:** Only eat organic meat, vegetables, and drink water

Meal 1

_____
_____
_____
_____

Meal 2

_____
_____
_____
_____

Meal 3

_____
_____
_____
_____

Meal 1

_____
_____
_____
_____
_____
_____
_____
_____
_____
_____
_____
_____
_____
_____
_____
_____
_____
_____
_____
_____

# CARDIO FOR 45 MINUTES

**30**DAY HUB Habit-Changing Challenge

Today's Date: _____ / _____ / _____

**Day 20:** Only eat organic meat, vegetables, and drink water

Meal 1

_____
_____
_____
_____

Meal 2

_____
_____
_____
_____

Meal 3

_____
_____
_____
_____

Meal 1

_____
_____
_____
_____
_____
_____
_____
_____
_____
_____
_____
_____
_____
_____
_____
_____
_____
_____
_____

| EXERCISE | SET #1 | SET #2 | SET #3 | SET #4 | SET #5 |
|---|---|---|---|---|---|
| Leg Extensions | | | | | |
| Squat | | | | | |
| Leg Press | | | | | |
| Leg Curl | | | | | |
| Lunge - Barbell/DB/Static/Step Up | | | | | |
| Leg Extensions | | | | | |

**30**DAY HUB Habit-Changing Challenge

Today's Date: _____ / _____ / _____

**Day 21:** Only eat organic meat, vegetables, and drink water

Meal 1

_____
_____
_____
_____

Meal 1

_____
_____
_____
_____
_____
_____
_____

Meal 2

_____
_____
_____
_____

_____
_____
_____
_____
_____
_____
_____

Meal 3

_____
_____
_____
_____

_____
_____
_____
_____

# CARDIO FOR 45 MINUTES

30DAY HUB Habit-Changing Challenge

Today's Date: _____ / _____ / _____

Meal 1

_____
_____
_____
_____

Meal 2

_____
_____
_____
_____

Meal 3

_____
_____
_____
_____

Meal 1

_____
_____
_____
_____
_____
_____
_____
_____
_____
_____
_____
_____
_____
_____
_____
_____

| EXERCISE | SET #1 | SET #2 | SET #3 | SET #4 |
|---|---|---|---|---|
| Incl. Flyes - Dumbbell | x10 | x10 | x10 | x10 |
| DB incline Bench Press | x10 | x10 | x10 | x10 |
| Machine Bench Press | x15 | x15 | x15 | x15 |
| Tricep "ARM" Extension | x15 | x15 | x15 | |
| Tricep Dumbbell Kickback | x20 | x20 | x20 | x20 |
| Overhead Press | x20 | x20 | x20 | x20 |
| Dumbbell Lateral Raises | x10 | x10 | x10 | x10 |
| Dumbbell Front Raise | x10 | x10 | x10 | x10 |
| High Pull | x10 | x10 | x10 | x10 |

**30**DAY HUB Habit-Changing Challenge

Today's Date: _____ / _____ / _____

**Day 23:** Only eat organic meat, vegetables, and drink water

Meal 1

_____
_____
_____
_____

Meal 2

_____
_____
_____
_____

Meal 3

_____
_____
_____
_____

Meal 1

_____
_____
_____
_____
_____
_____
_____
_____
_____
_____
_____
_____
_____
_____
_____
_____
_____
_____
_____

# CARDIO FOR 45 MINUTES

**30**DAY HUB Habit-Changing Challenge

Today's Date: _____ / _____ / _____

**Day 24:** Only eat organic meat, vegetables, and drink water

Meal 1
_____
_____
_____
_____

Meal 2
_____
_____
_____
_____

Meal 3
_____
_____
_____
_____

Meal 1
_____
_____
_____
_____
_____
_____
_____
_____
_____
_____
_____
_____
_____
_____
_____
_____

| EXERCISE | SET #1 | SET #2 | SET #3 | SET #4 | SET #5 |
|---|---|---|---|---|---|
| Pulldowns - Wide Grip & Narrow Grip | x20 | x20 | x20 | x20 | |
| Seated Row | x15 | x15 | x15 | x15 | |
| Bent "Dumbbell" Row | x20 | x20 | x20 | x20 | |
| Machine Bicep Curl | x15 | x15 | x15 | | |
| Standing Barbell Curl | x10 | x10 | x10 | x10 | |
| Seated Alternating Dumbbell Curl | x20 | x20 | x20 | x20 | |

**30**DAY HUB Habit-Changing Challenge

Today's Date: _____ / _____ / _____

Meal 1

_____
_____
_____
_____

Meal 1

_____
_____
_____
_____
_____
_____
_____
_____

Meal 2

_____
_____
_____
_____

_____
_____
_____
_____
_____
_____
_____

Meal 3

_____
_____
_____
_____

_____
_____
_____
_____
_____

# CARDIO FOR 45 MINUTES

**30**DAY HUB Habit-Changing Challenge

Today's Date: _____ / _____ / _____

**Day 26:** Only eat organic meat, vegetables, and drink water

Meal 1

_____
_____
_____
_____

Meal 2

_____
_____
_____
_____

Meal 3

_____
_____
_____
_____

Meal 1

_____
_____
_____
_____
_____
_____
_____
_____
_____
_____
_____
_____
_____
_____
_____
_____
_____
_____
_____
_____

| EXERCISE | SET #1 | SET #2 | SET #3 | SET #4 | SET #5 |
|---|---|---|---|---|---|
| Leg Extensions | | | | | |
| Squat | | | | | |
| Leg Press | | | | | |
| Leg Curl | | | | | |
| Lunge - Barbell/DB/Static/Step Up | | | | | |
| Leg Extensions | | | | | |

Today's Date: _____ / _____ / _____

**30**DAY HUB Habit-Changing Challenge

**Day 27:** Only eat organic meat, vegetables, and drink water

Meal 1

_____
_____
_____
_____

Meal 2

_____
_____
_____
_____

Meal 3

_____
_____
_____
_____

Meal 1

_____
_____
_____
_____
_____
_____
_____
_____
_____
_____
_____
_____
_____
_____
_____
_____
_____
_____

# CARDIO FOR 45 MINUTES

**30**DAY HUB Habit-Changing Challenge

Today's Date: _____ / _____ / _____

# Day 28: Only eat organic meat, vegetables, and drink water

Meal 1

_____

_____

_____

_____

Meal 2

_____

_____

_____

_____

Meal 3

_____

_____

_____

_____

Meal 1

_____

_____

_____

_____

_____

_____

_____

_____

_____

_____

_____

_____

_____

_____

_____

_____

_____

_____

| EXERCISE | SET #1 | SET #2 | SET #3 | SET #4 |
|---|---|---|---|---|
| Incl. Flyes - Dumbbell | x10 | x10 | x10 | x10 |
| DB incline Bench Press | x10 | x10 | x10 | x10 |
| Machine Bench Press | x15 | x15 | x15 | x15 |
| Tricep "ARM" Extension | x15 | x15 | x15 | |
| Tricep Dumbbell Kickback | x20 | x20 | x20 | x20 |
| Overhead Press | x20 | x20 | x20 | x20 |
| Dumbbell Lateral Raises | x10 | x10 | x10 | x10 |
| Dumbbell Front Raise | x10 | x10 | x10 | x10 |
| High Pull | x10 | x10 | x10 | x10 |

**30**DAY HUB Habit-Changing Challenge

Today's Date: _____ / _____ / _____

**Day 29:** Only eat organic meat, vegetables, and drink water

Meal 1
_____
_____
_____
_____

Meal 2
_____
_____
_____
_____

Meal 3
_____
_____
_____
_____

Meal 1
_____
_____
_____
_____
_____
_____
_____
_____
_____
_____
_____
_____
_____
_____
_____
_____
_____
_____
_____
_____

# CARDIO FOR 45 MINUTES

30DAY HUB Habit-Changing Challenge

Today's Date: _____ / _____ / _____

# Day 30: Only eat organic meat, vegetables, and drink water

Meal 1

_____
_____
_____
_____

Meal 2

_____
_____
_____
_____

Meal 3

_____
_____
_____
_____

Meal 1

_____
_____
_____
_____
_____
_____
_____
_____
_____
_____
_____
_____
_____
_____
_____
_____
_____
_____
_____
_____

| EXERCISE | SET #1 | SET #2 | SET #3 | SET #4 | SET #5 |
|---|---|---|---|---|---|
| Pulldowns - Wide Grip & Narrow Grip | x20 | x20 | x20 | x20 | |
| Seated Row | x15 | x15 | x15 | x15 | |
| Bent "Dumbbell" Row | x20 | x20 | x20 | x20 | |
| Machine Bicep Curl | x15 | x15 | x15 | | |
| Standing Barbell Curl | x10 | x10 | x10 | x10 | |
| Seated Alternating Dumbbell Curl | x20 | x20 | x20 | x20 | |

**30**DAY HUB Habit-Changing Challenge

Today's Date: _____ / _____ / _____

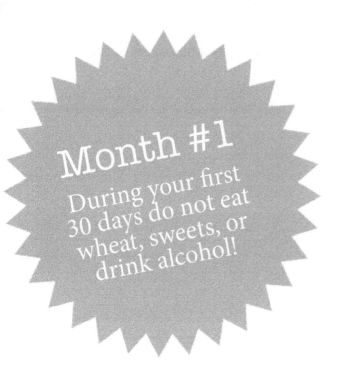

Month #1

During your first 30 days do not eat wheat, sweets, or drink alcohol!

"The chains of habit are too light to be felt until they are too heavy to be broken."
- Warren Buffett
(The legendary investor worth $89.2 billion as of May 2019)

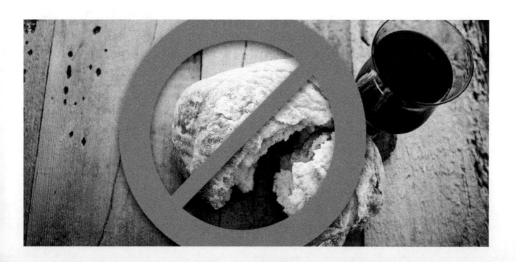

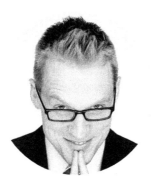

"I'm starting to feel like Luke wants you
and I to only eat organic meat, organic
vegetables, and to drink water."
- Clay Clark
(Contributing writer for Forbes, founder of
DJConnection.com, co-founder of EITRLounge.
com, founder of EpicPhotos.com, founder of
MakeYourLifeEpic.com, etc.)

# Chapter 3
## The Fitness Plan

"It's not what we do once in a while
that shapes our lives. It's what we do
consistently."
- Tony Robbins

(The New York Times best-selling author, entrepreneur,
philanthropist and life coach. He is most well known for
his powerful self help seminars and books, including
*Awake the Giant Within* and *Unlimited Power*)

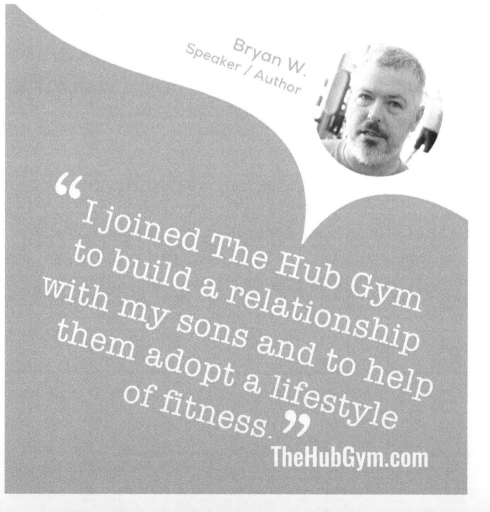

Bryan W.
Speaker / Author

"I joined The Hub Gym
to build a relationship
with my sons and to help
them adopt a lifestyle
of fitness."

TheHubGym.com

# BODY MEASUREMENTS
## HEIGHT

(Learn more about this chart on page 50)

FEET

_____

INCHES

_____

| DATE: | | | | | | | | |
|---|---|---|---|---|---|---|---|---|
| WEIGHT | | | | | | | | |
| BICEPS | | | | | | | | |
| WAIST (BELLY BUTTON) | | | | | | | | |
| SHOULDERS | | | | | | | | |
| CHEST | | | | | | | | |
| THIGHS | | | | | | | | |
| CALVES | | | | | | | | |

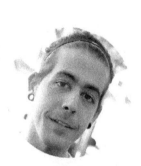

Colton E.
Hub Member Services

" The Hub Gym has a very warm and inviting family atmosphere. "

TheHubGym.com

## Track Your Progress and Goals

The chart below can be somewhat daunting, but I promise if you do not do it now you will regret it in four weeks when things start changing. Over the years, I have found that even though recording measurements is not the most fun thing to do the clients that do track their results are always amazed at the changes they make. Recording your progress is also a way of keeping your goals at the forefront of your mind when you start having negative self-talk or think about abandoning your goals. I suggest updating this chart every month and then don't worry about these numbers more than once per month. Let how you feel and how your clothes are fitting your body be the measuring stick for your progress. Take notice of how your body is changing, or not, and then we can alter your plan to compliment these changes. In addition to the chart, I would highly recommend taking "before" pictures of yourself because then you'll be able to see where you are starting, and as you take progress pics (once a month) you can see real results in real time.

The foundation of success in the world of fitness is a plan that is well prepared and easy to follow. Below are the proven tools that will help you kick-start your fitness journey.

The simple act of moving your body often enough will help you regain control of your health and fitness. A quick walk around the block or a session in the gym can release endorphins that will give you the energy to keep going. As your energy increases you will naturally begin doing more and thereby realize more results. The first step is generally the hardest to take but, trust me, once you make the decision to take that first step you will start living your best life.

**The 5 W's of Fitness Success**

1. What?

What is it that you hope to achieve? And what has been the biggest barrier for you when it comes to your health and fitness goals?

_____
_____

_____
_____


2. Where?

Where would you like to see yourself in one month, three months, six months and one year?

_____
_____

_____
_____

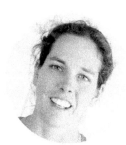

Yoga Instructor / Teacher
Lexi A.

" I love the personal
feel of The Hub Gym.
It feels like my gym. "

TheHubGym.com

## 3. When?

When will you work out throughout the week? There has to be time specifically set aside for your workout. Put it on the calendar today.

_____

_____

_____

## 4. Who?

Who is going to benefit the most by you choosing to invest in your health?

_____

_____

_____

## 5. Winning! Winners take steps to be better, and you've taken a first step. You are a winner.

Share your early wins here, no matter how small.

_____

_____

_____

**Don't Be Intimidated by the Gym. Move Your Body.**

I have found that the biggest barrier for people after joining a gym is that they have no idea what to do with the equipment in the facility. With this hurdle in mind, my goal was to create workout logs that cover the major muscle groups in a simple-to-follow format. There are three separate logs - each one represents a major muscle group and are a great mix of free weight exercises as well as machine exercises. My team of fitness coaches will take you through these workouts during your first step assessment to ensure you feel equipped to execute them on your own. Our first step assessment is the time where one of our professional fitness coaches meets with new clients like you to help you find the right path to get into the best shape of your life.

It's at this time that we determine what The Hub Gym team and facility can also do to help you accomplish your fitness goals. We have had thousands of clients make amazing progress going through our first step assessment and using these workout logs, so make sure you schedule your first step assessment to learn how to most effectively put these logs to work for you.

**Here's the basic breakdown of what a week of training will look like:**

- Strength training three days a week, one hour per session (Use the workout logs provided)
- High-intensity interval training one day a week (participate in the wide variety of group fitness classes offered with your membership)
- Steady-state cardio one day a week, 35 to 45 minutes per session (treadmill, bike, go for a walk)
- Two days of active recovery

The next time you find yourself feeling down, tired or just plain worn out put on your walking shoes and take a nice walk around the block. Notice as you are taking in the fresh air how your mood is elevated and by the time you are back at your front door you'll feel like a different person. Sure, that hill in your neighborhood causes your lungs and legs to burn but the sense of accomplishment resembles that of Rocky Balboa at the top of the stairs and you almost start screaming "Adrian, I did it!" But the truth of the matter is that you did do it!

That simple act is all that is required to change your life if you will just commit to doing it on a consistent basis. You must put your workouts into your calendar and daily schedule or you won't do it. The road to fitness doesn't have to be grueling and unpleasant, it just has to be consistent. My goal at The Hub Gym is to provide you with a safe place, a team of people to help you structure a plan of success, and then offer the accountability you need to stay consistent. Now it's up to you to decide what you want, and do not stop until you achieve it.

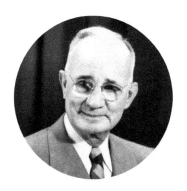

"Action is the real measure of intelligence."
- Napoleon Hill

(Best-selling author of *Think and Grow Rich*)

# Chapter 4 My Story

"Your life does not get better by chance, it gets better by change."
- Jim Rohn
(The famous entrepreneur, author and motivational speaker)

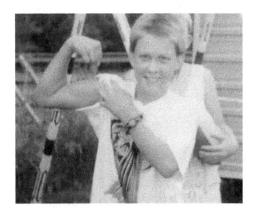

**Luke as a Youngster**

After completing a degree in Visual Communications and Graphic Design I found myself working a regular nine-to-five job with people who had literally been sitting in the same desk for decades doing the same tasks every day. I did my best to liven the place up and to make a positive impact on the lives of those I worked around, but I quickly realized the box I was living in was only so big and my exposure to new experiences and people was limited. I worked a few more years in the field

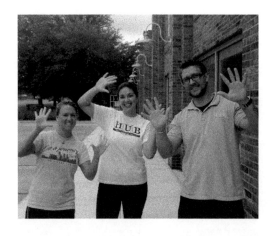

until one night I was sitting in a small group being asked the question "If you didn't have to do what you are doing today what would you do?"

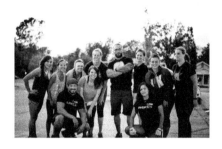

That question hit me like a ton of bricks and I realized a change was necessary. While I didn't have a specific job or career path as an answer I did know I wanted to be around as many people as possible and that I wanted to help those people to continually grow and change. In that same small group there was a guy whose father had started a gym franchise and wanted to sell a few of their locations. A month or so later I was the proud owner of a small gym in Broken Arrow, Oklahoma.

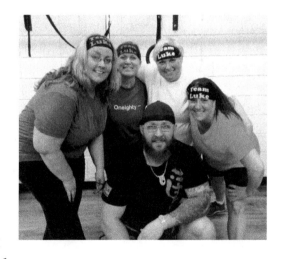

Immediately, I had access to a constantly-changing atmosphere and group of people but also the reality that I had just purchased a business that was not able to pay for my current humble and financially frugal lifestyle. For the next six years I grinded it out and built an amazing community of people and eventually, in 2011, I was able to rebrand our original gym into The Hub Gym and move it to our current location in the Rose District on Main Street in Broken Arrow. Through a lot of trial and error and hard work, The Hub is now thriving, and my dream has finally become a reality.

During this transition I learned tons of valuable lessons about what it truly takes to run a business and how to build quality relationships. We are now nearly eight years into this new journey we call The Hub Gym. While the path has at times been rough I can honestly say I am proud of what we have built. We are now truly serving our community and great people like you.

My story is a true reflection of what it takes to make any other story a success. All that is required is for one to get honest, to decide you want to succeed, and surround yourself with people who have the answers you need and someone to hold you accountable if you can't hold yourself accountable. There is not some magical potion that some people have and others don't. It is literally dependent on your choices and your ownership of those choices.

My hope is that The Hub Gym and I can continue to inspire our members and community about what is possible when ordinary people make a choice to turn their dreams into reality.

**Fact:** According to the center for Disease Control and Prevention Data from 2015-2016 shows that nearly 1 in 5 school age children and young people (6-19 years) in the united states struggles with obesity.

In the United States, the percentage of children & adolescents affected by obesity has nearly tripled since the 1970s.

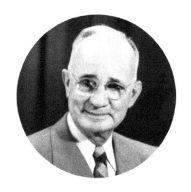

"The time will never be just right, you must
act now."
- Napoleon Hill
(Best-selling author of *Think and Grow Rich*)

"A journey of a thousand miles begins with a
single step."
- Chinese Proverbs

# Chapter 5
## Change is Possible - Retrain Your Brain to Believe It

"Change your thoughts and you change your world."
- Norman Vincent Peale
(The best selling author of *The Power of Positive Thinking*.)

It's likely when you walked into The Hub Gym it wasn't your first trip to a gym, nor will it be your last step toward losing weight or getting healthy and becoming healthier. The truth is, changing our habits is an uphill challenge for many of us. In fact, many of us have been making the same choices and implementing the same routines for most of our lives, so shaking things up can be downright uncomfortable. Just walking into a gym is a test of strength for some of us. And while the act of walking through the gym doors is a small success,

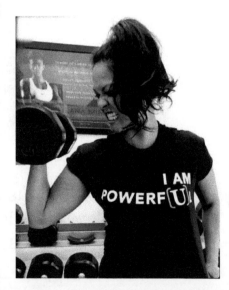

Eve Peppers showing us "She is Powerful"

it will ultimately come down to the daily action steps that you commit to taking that will determine whether you actually achieve your goals or not. Quite honestly, fitness success doesn't start with the gym, with your fabulous new workout gear, or the latest supplement, it starts with reorganizing your schedule and changing your habits.

In order to achieve the results that you may have been seeking for years or months you must first remove the limiting beliefs which have played a huge role in getting you where you are today. The primary limiting factor in most people's fitness

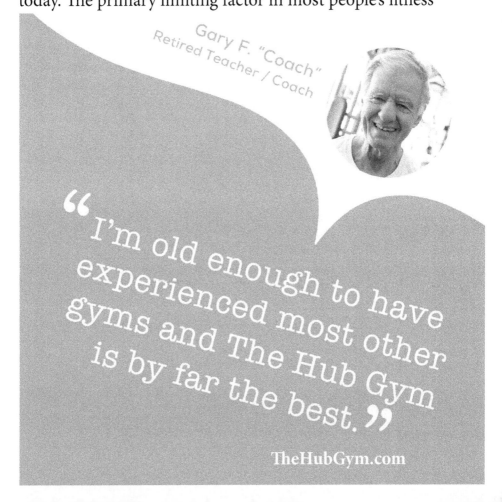

Gary F. "Coach"
Retired Teacher / Coach

"I'm old enough to have experienced most other gyms and The Hub Gym is by far the best."

TheHubGym.com

journey is the belief that "I am past the point of return so I may as well not even try." With this being the loudest and most predominant voice in our heads it is no wonder that the Huffington Post reports that only 8% of people will actually keep their New Year's resolutions.

What you tell yourself and how you speak to yourself is the deciding factor in your personal transformation.

It's important to remember this. Your thoughts create your feelings which in turn create your actions, and your actions

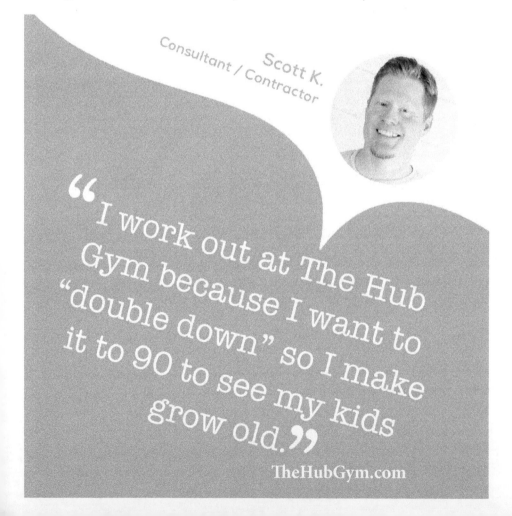

Consultant / Contractor    Scott K.

"I work out at The Hub Gym because I want to "double down" so I make it to 90 to see my kids grow old."

TheHubGym.com

(what you do every day) create your life. Often times we live such busy lives, filled with constant distraction and we never take the time needed to ask ourselves what is causing our current realty. My friend, if you and I are not careful we

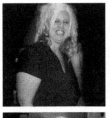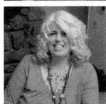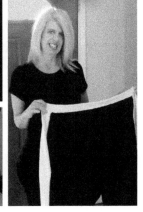

can live life in a habitually dysfunctional autopilot mode. If we allow our emotions to take the reigns, and we just continue to make the same poor decisions over and over as our subconscious minds are always looking for the easiest way to get through life.

*Michelle H. - Transformation*

So what can be done? How can you move to living the purpose-driven life of your dreams? You must decide today that you are going to block out time in your schedule for working out. In order to get in the best shape of your life you must choose what thoughts you are going to allow yourself to think.

Do not allow your past failures to become the roadblocks in the way of your future success. Every single moment is a new opportunity to make better decisions, and a new opportunity to align yourself with the mindset needed to become the best version of your future self.

**Let's start with working out.**

Your path to physical fitness success is guaranteed when you follow a proven path. By developing specific, measurable, actionable, realistic, and time-sensetive goals, you will achieve success. Taking these intentional first steps will allow you to take control of your health and to avoid the things that have derailed you up to this point in your life.

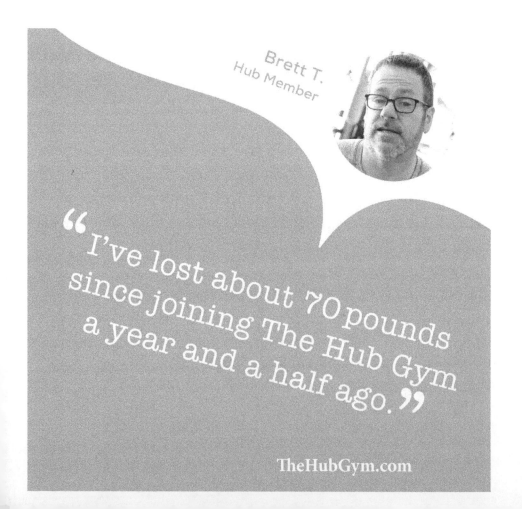

Brett T.
Hub Member

"I've lost about 70 pounds since joining The Hub Gym a year and a half ago."

TheHubGym.com

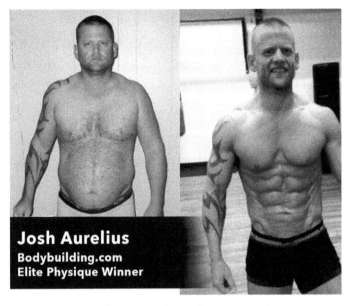

**Josh Aurelius**
Bodybuilding.com
Elite Physique Winner

*Josh A. - Transformation*

Over the years, I have discovered new members' primary emotion is fear or frustration for where they are in regards to their overall health and overall body image. Through our first step assessment there is an opportunity for you to voice these fears and then we ask for you to trust us to show you the proven path.

In that moment of trust and vulnerability you will see a shift and a spark of hope. Over the years thousands have chosen to be brave and to trust our team, and the process.

During the first few years after I started The Hub Gym I met thousands of great people sign up for a gym membership only to quit a few months later because they were not seeing the results they wanted to see. They were paying a small monthly fee for a gym membership but they would not show up, and then a few months later they would quit.

In order to help great people like you get the fitness results you are seeking I worked with my team to create what I now call the first step assessment. Since implementing the first step assessment there have been countless success stories where people like you have met or exceeded their fitness goals. One story in particular that really sticks out to me is the story of a mother who came into our gym very nervous and apprehensive of even walking in. She came into our gym during the hottest time of the summer in a full sweat suit with the look of desperation on her face.

After a long conversation with a member of our team she decided to take the plunge and trust our staff to coach her along the journey. She has now been a member for more than six years and has lost well over 160 pounds. We will never forget the day she walked in and told us, "My son hugged me today and said Mom this is the first time I have been able to put my arms all the way around you." This is one of many stories of its kind but it absolutely touches our hearts every time we see her.

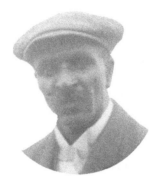

"99% of failures come from people who have
the habit of
making excuses."
- George Washington Carver
(Famous American botonist and inventor who was born
a slave)

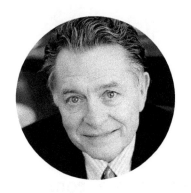

"One of the main reasons people don't
improve is that they are not honest with
themselves."
- Lee Cockerell
(Former executive Vice President of Walt Disney World
Resorts who once managed 40,000 employees and
1,000,000 customers per week)

# Chapter 6
## Because We Care

"There is no passion to be found playing small and in settling for a life that is less than the one you are capable of living."
- Nelson Mandela

(Nelson Mandela was the first democratically elected president of South Africa, as well as the first black president of the nation. He spent nearly three decades in prison for his anti-apartheid views and for organizing peaceful protests.)

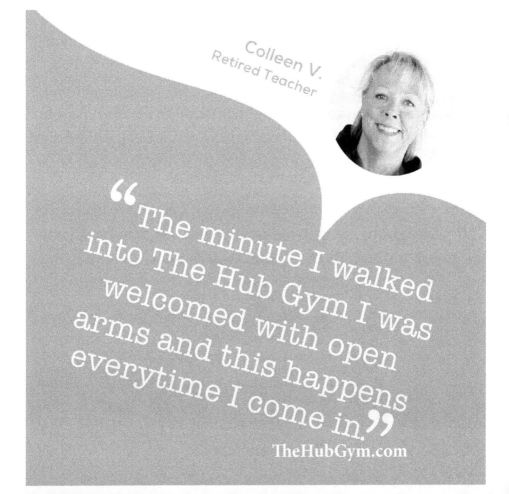

Colleen V.
Retired Teacher

"The minute I walked into The Hub Gym I was welcomed with open arms and this happens everytime I come in."

TheHubGym.com

## What Makes The Hub Gym Different From Most Gyms?

We want to get to know who you are and what you hope to achieve by investing in your physical fitness. We know that for most people going to the gym is not the most enjoyable experience (it's not a theme park, mall, etc). A gym is a place where people really dig deep and are coming face to face with things they don't like about themselves. We truly care, and want to join you on your journey.

I think my level of care comes from realizing I am where I am today because of the people who cared enough for me to be a light in my life. At a base level, we as humans are here to build community and walk with each other through life. For me, our members are an extension of our family and it is such a blessing to see people realize their goals and to be living their best lives.

I receive as much if not more from the people we are in contact with. I learn from being in fellowship with our members, I am able to live my best life by serving great members like you.

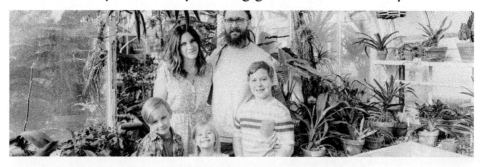

*The Owens Family*

## The Facility

Thank goodness for my wife, Lily. She helped ensure the atmosphere of The Hub Gym was unlike any other gym. I wanted hardcore music, chalk dust flying in the air and super masculine colors that reflected who I was at the time. Fortunately, Lily had a brighter vision for The Hub and for me. What you will find when you come into The Hub is a very eclectic, easy going atmosphere where anyone should feel right at home, our gym is open 24/7 and the colors in the gym are light and uplifting. Today our facility features amazing hardwood ceilings and a bank of floor-to-ceiling windows that allow for natural light to fill the space.

Although we are a more intimate & small boutique facility, when working out at the Hub Gym you will have access to a full line of cardio and strength training equipment, group fitness classes, showers, and spacious locker rooms.

## The Environment

We pride ourselves in creating and maintaining an environment where everyone feels at home. It doesn't matter if you have been in the gym your whole life or just stepped foot in the gym for your first time, you will not feel intimidated or out of place. The Hub attracts a wide variety of people, and we welcome everyone. We have a lot of men and women who love our group fitness classes, families who enjoy our friendly and welcoming atmosphere, but we also have serious workout folks who love our gym because they want a deadlift platform and heavy weights. Our members like to train at The Hub because it's like being part of a family. You meet people and build relationships inside The Hub that continues outside the gym, and it definitely makes going to the gym something to look forward to.

## Our Staff

We are very intentional in who we allow to be a part of The Hub team as we realize our team is a direct reflection of us as founders. We have implemented a rigorous hiring process which helps us to ensure our clients are in the best hands possible, and we are always recruiting happy and positive people to join our team.

## Training Designed for People Like You

It is our goal to ensure our clients are being coached by able and capable trainers. To provide you with the best experience possible our trainers are put through a rigorous hiring process whereby they must shadow current trainers and be coached in The Hub's approach to physical fitness.

## We Are Invested In Your Success

While each person is responsible for how they show up to this game called life, we at The Hub Gym know that with a bit of help our clients accomplish their fitness goals. Our first step assessment is our way of investing in you and giving you a platform of success to stand on throughout your journey. While the path, at times has been rough for me, I can honestly say I am proud of what we have built. We are now truly serving our community and great people like you the way I had always hoped we would.

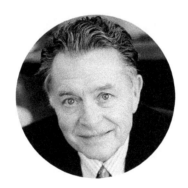

"One way to get priorities accomplished is to schedule them into your calendar."
- Lee Cockerell
(Former executive Vice President of Walt Disney World Resorts)

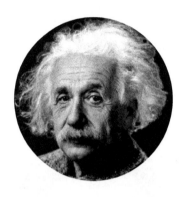

"Great spirits have encountered violent
opposition from
mediocre minds."
- Albert Einstein
(Renowned Theoretical Physicist)

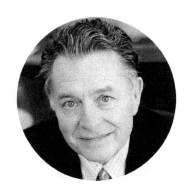

"You either pay now or pay later with just
about every decision you make about where
and how you spend your time."
- Lee Cockerell

(Former executive Vice President of Walt Disney World
Resorts)

# Chapter 7
# Why People (Not You) Don't Get Results

"If not now, when?"
- Eckhart Tolle
(Eckhart Tolle is a spiritual teacher. He is a German-
born resident of Canada best known as the author of
*The Power of Now* and *A New Earth: Awakening to Your
Life's Purpose.*)

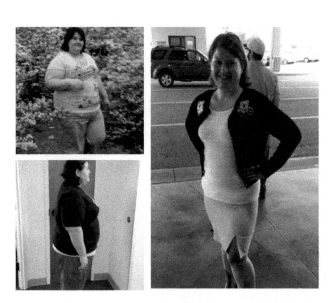

*Krystal S. - Transformation*

**If nothing changes, nothing will change.**

If you don't enjoy your current situation or are finding
your life just isn't working the
way you are doing it now, we are here to help you.
However, once we help you to identify the system or
process that does work it is best to keep doing what

works. So you need to be willing to change so that you are able to achieve your goals. You must stick to a path that has proven to be successful instead of following the next trend or get-fit-quick scheme.

## Lack of Commitment

It is possible to be committed to chaos and dysfunction which is why it is so important to surround yourself with people who have the things you are wanting out

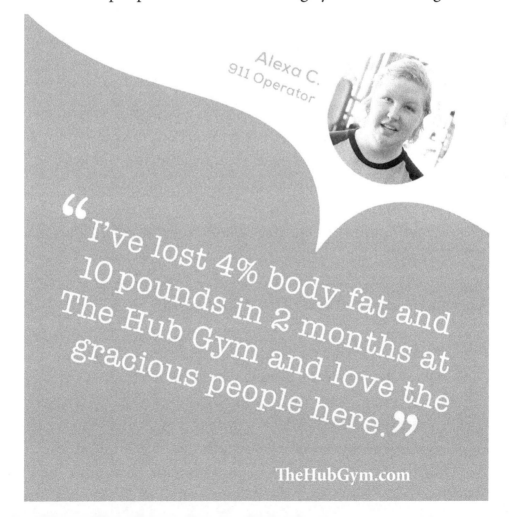

Alexa C.
911 Operator

"I've lost 4% body fat and 10 pounds in 2 months at The Hub Gym and love the gracious people here."

TheHubGym.com

of life and to stay committed to following the path and get the results you are looking for. All too often we get started down a path that is leading us to our dreams but as soon as most people encounter any adversity they quit. It is so much easier to stay the course than it is to create a whole new course. Our path and system is proven to be life-changing so stick it out and the results will come.

## Lack of Schedule/No Plan

Desire can often be the catalyst for change, but without a plan and direction your
desire can quickly turn into distress and destruction. We must match our desires with a plan and schedule that makes sense. Analyze your schedule and structure your plan in a way that is manageable and that will produce the greatest likelihood of your success. Intentions are great but a plan with a source of accountability is far more likely to produce the desired results.

## Unrealistic Expectations - How to Set a goal

Make sure your goals are realistic for your current situation. A great example would be if you are coming into your fitness journey having never worked out and weighing 350 pounds it is probably unrealistic to think you are going to have a six pack and run a marathon within a month. What is more realistic is committing to coming to the gym or doing some form of exercise 3-5 times per week and making water your only source of hydration in your first month. As long as you realize you have now chosen a lifestyle of fitness that first month will be an amazing success and if this doesn't feel like success you need to dig a bit deeper to find the reason why you are pursuing fitness in the first place. It has to be about you and your desires and not about making someone else happy or for any other external reason.

**How to Set Realistic Goals**

Our team has helped thousands of people to identify what their realistic goals are, and we're committed to sticking with you through your journey. The best way to identify your success plan is to schedule your free personalized first step program with one of our fitness coaches.

We find our clients that schedule their first step assessment come away with an arsenal of tools and a new perspective. They realize the requirements for drastic change are all within their power and the only prerequisite is to make the decision to stick to the plan and to get back on the plan when they fall off the path.

## How The Hub Makes this Hurdle Easy for People

The staff at The Hub does a great job of keeping a finger on the pulse of our members which helps ensure our members don't spend too much time "off the path".

We have created a culture of accountability which provides our active members with the path to run on for continual progress.

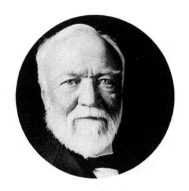

"People who are unable to motivate themselves must be content with mediocrity, no matter how impressive their other talents."
- Andrew Carnegie
(World's wealthiest man during his lifetime who began working at the age of just 13)

# Chapter 8

# Our History

"You need an attitude of service. You're not just serving yourself. You help others to grow up and you grow with them."
- David Green
(The founder and CEO of Hobby Lobby, a chain of arts and crafts stores. He opened his first store in 1970 with a $600 loan, today Hobby Lobby does $3.3 billion in sales.)

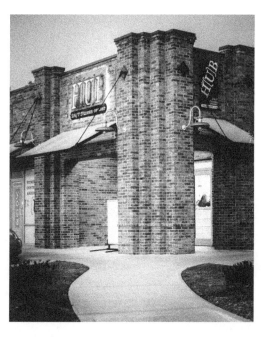

We know a thing or two about transformations - not only for our members, but the very building we dwell in. Originally, in the 1950s, the building was a Humpty Dumpty Supermarket, and then it became a Farmers Coop where you could buy sacks of animal feed and live baby chicks. When the Farmers Coop moved out, the building remained empty for years and became a dilapidated eyesore, before it was purchased in 2007 by my father and mother in law, Jim and Pat Bomar. Just like a person's body that's been ignored for years, we weren't giving up on this old building. We saw its bones, the history, the potential, what it could be with a lot of love and attention. After much work and dedication the new building was finished and we opened The Hub Gym doors in September 2011.

As one of the very first new business shopping centers in the Rose District of Broken Arrow, most people thought we were crazy to invest in an undeveloped part of Broken Arrow but we saw the potential for this location allowing us to become the "Cheers" of the new district and community. At The Hub we have a saying, it's kind of hokey but it's how we truly feel: "We don't have members, we have friendbers." We like to get to know

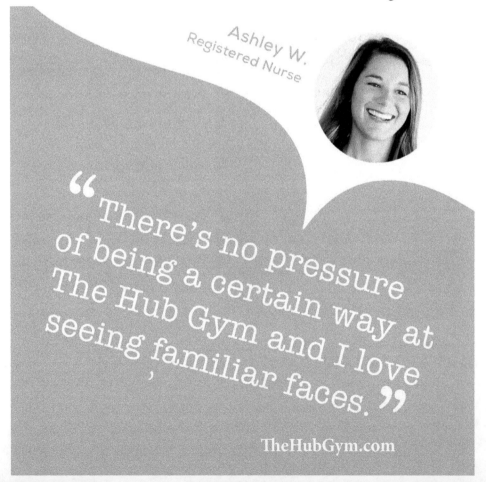

Ashley W.
Registered Nurse

"There's no pressure of being a certain way at The Hub Gym and I love seeing familiar faces."

TheHubGym.com

our members, help them feel comfortable, and love to invest in their fitness journey. As The Hub Gym becomes a place our members look forward to coming to, and not someplace they dread. More and more physical transformations are occurring. The Hub is more than a gym. It's an experience.

The heart behind The Hub has always been service. Service to our members and the community. It is our goal to create a fun, safe and productive atmosphere whereby the members and surrounding community have the opportunity to become the very best version of themselves. That's why we named it The Hub Gym in the first place. After much searching and many hours of discussion we honed in on the name "The Hub" because it was important to us to be the center of health, fitness, and community within Broken Arrow. A hub for activity. The very structure of the word compliments our mission "Fitness Centered Around You" in that the [U] is at the center of the word. The well-being of our members has always been at the core of our focus.
We're not a big-box gym, and we don't want to be. Therefore there will always be some things we can't compete with the chain gyms on. We understand this, and we just focus on being the best Hub we can be. And it's paying off. The HUB has been voted number one fitness center and athletic center year after year now in Broken Arrow competing against -> 10 Gym, Genesis, Planet Fitness, Sky Fitness, as well as Gym of the Month on Bodybuilding.com. And we're just getting started.

The Hub Gym exists because of my passion for helping people make a difference in their lives. I want The Hub to be a place where you can exhale from the day's stresses, to be encouraged, and to be reminded of your own power. At the Hub Gym you're not just a member; you're part of The Hub family. Welcome, we can't wait to get to know you.

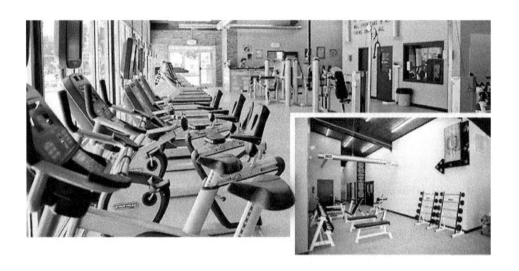

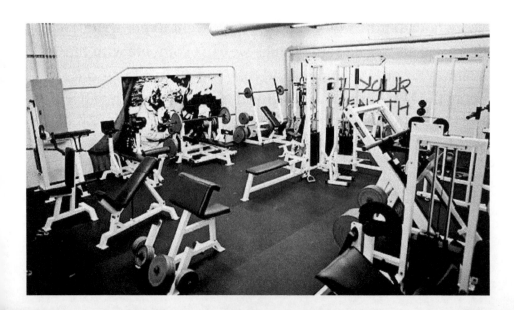

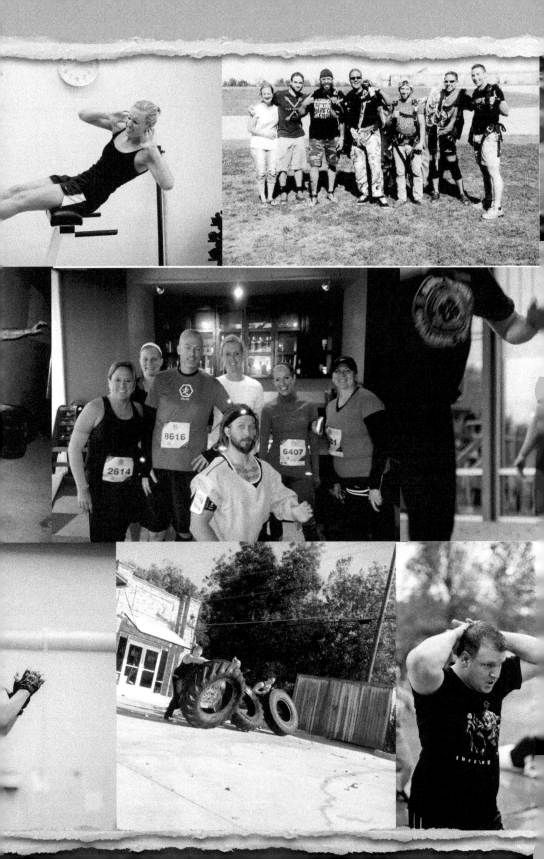

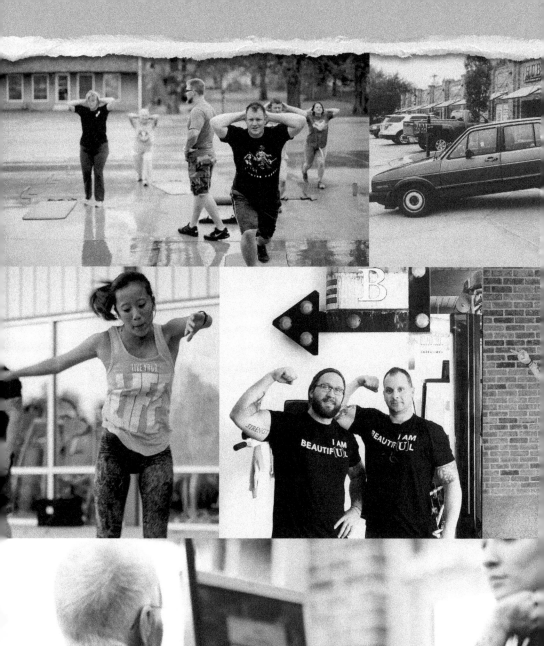

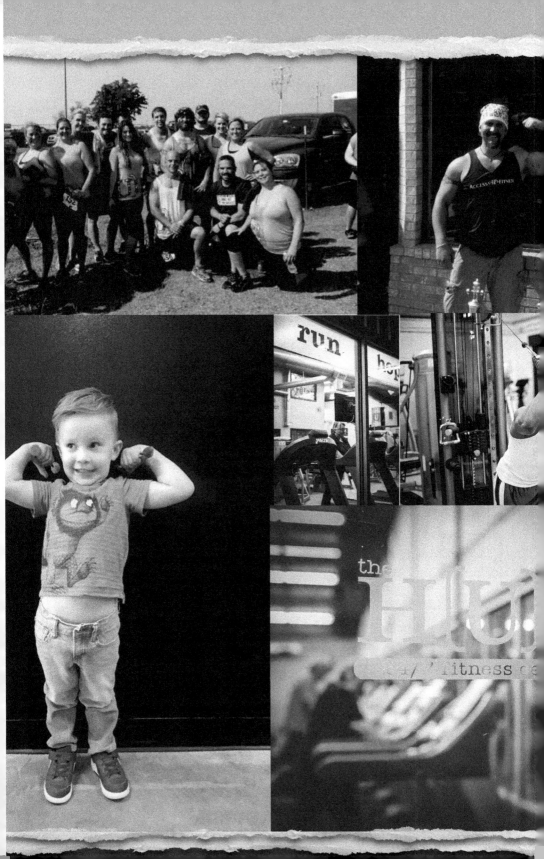

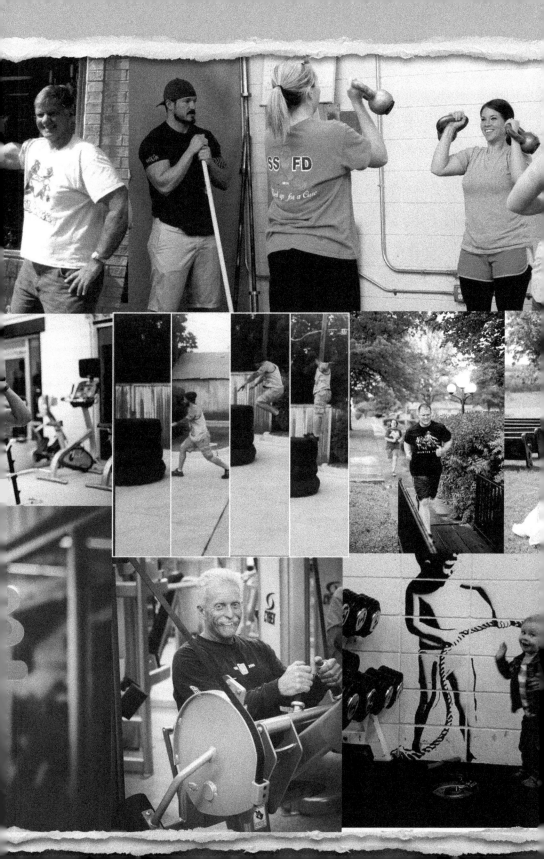

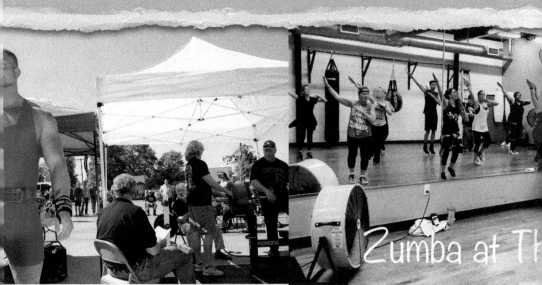

Zumba at Th

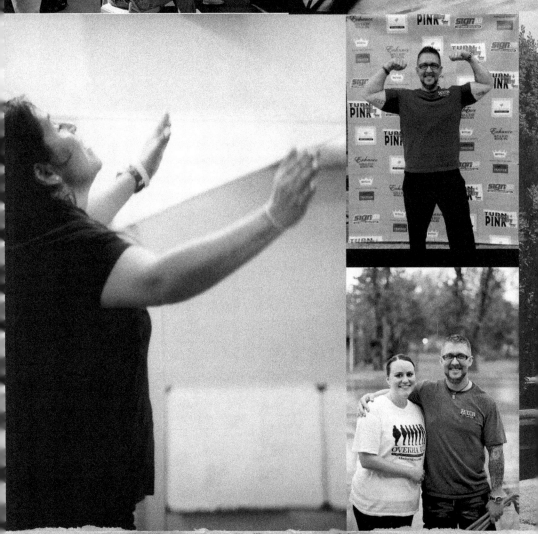

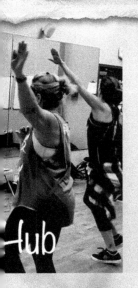

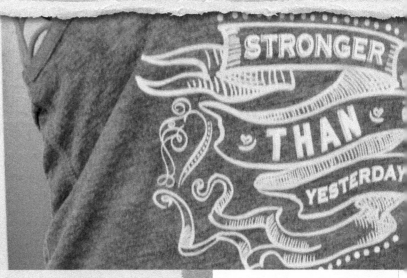

STRONGER
THAN
YESTERDAY

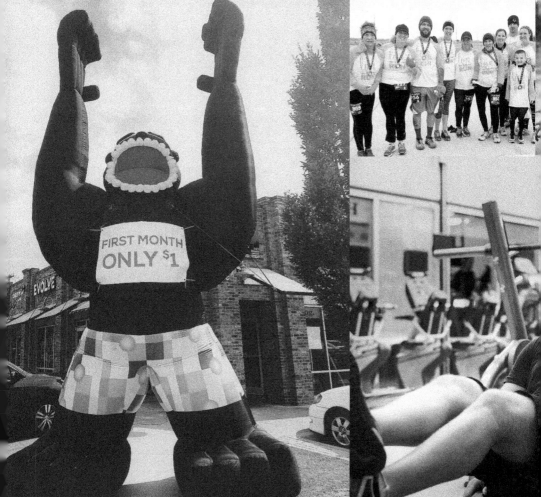

FIRST MONTH
ONLY $1